Reverse Hypertension
Lower your high blood pressure with simple steps

Dr. Shahriar Mostafa

MBBS, MPH

Copyright 2017 Dr. Shahriar Mostafa

This ebook is licensed for your personal enjoyment only. This ebook may not be resold or reproduce in any format without written permission of the author. Thank you for respecting the hard work of this author.

Introduction

Let's have the bad news first.

Hypertension or high blood pressure is the number one killer worldwide. It is a disease of pandemic proportion, affecting more and more people worldwide. Hypertension is the number one cause of heart attack and stroke, and it's poorly controlled worldwide.

Recent World Health Report by World Health Organization (WHO) gives us an alarming information, it says "Overall, approximately 20% of the world's adults are estimated to have hypertension. The prevalence dramatically increases in patients older than 60 years: In many countries, 50% of individuals in this age group (60+) have hypertension. Worldwide, approximately 1 billion people have hypertension, contributing to more than 7.1 million deaths per year".

Now the good news.

Hypertension or high blood pressure is very easy to keep in control. And with proper control, it's a normal condition. You don't need expensive programs, a lot of medicine or a big chunk of your time to keep hypertension in check. Following a simple routine can make it possible.

Before we begin few important things, you need to know.

Your interest in this book indicates that most likely you or your spouse or a family member has hypertension. Or you may want to prevent hypertension. So, it's possible that you have read and researched the internet about the condition and already know some of the information this book provide. But there is some new information which you will learn and this book will refresh what you know with latest data.

Another aspect of this book is, it is a small book. Our life has become very busy. We are connected all the time. With so much to see, learn and share we are always in short of time. It is difficult, sometimes unnecessary and time-consuming to read a long book crammed with useless information or search the internet for hours for information on blood pressure. This small book is packed with information that you will really need day to day. It is designed to save you a lot of time searching information on hypertension.

Now a few words about me. By profession, I am a doctor, completed my medical school 8 years back. Then I did a master's degree in public health (MPH). I have been working in a medical college hospital, treating patients and working on disease prevention for last 7 years. I write patient education books on diseases more than a year now, thanks to you I have two Amazon bestselling books. Writing on diseases gives me the opportunity to reach a broad audience, it gives me a chance to work on disease prevention on a larger scale.

Enough about me now let's begin to control hypertension.

IMPORTANT

I have another book on hypertension **"High Blood Pressure: Control with and Without Medicine"** available in Amazon. The content of this book is similar due to similar subject. Keep in mind that if you have purchased **"High Blood Pressure: Control with and Without Medicine"** then you don't need to buy this book.

You may buy **"High Blood Pressure: Control with and Without Medicine"** with or after buying this book, as it contains more detailed information on hypertension.

Table of Contents

Introduction 2
Notes 8
Hypertension or High blood pressure. 10
Risk factors for developing high blood pressure 13
Cause of High Blood Pressure 16
Symptoms of Hypertension 22
Diagnosis of Hypertension 24
Problems with uncontrolled hypertension 26
Treatment Options for High Blood Pressure 28
    Prehypertension 29
    Stage 1 Hypertension 32
    Stage 2 Hypertension 33
    Stage 3 Hypertension 34
Medicines used in Hypertension 36
    Diuretics 39
    Beta-Blockers 41
    Alpha-blockers for Hypertension 42
    ACE inhibitors 44
    Calcium Channel Blockers 46
    Angiotensin II Receptor Blockers (ARB) 46
    Direct Vasodilators 47
    Central Agonists 48
    Direct Renin Inhibitors 48
    Peripheral-Acting Adrenergic Blockers 49
Medicine for Specific Conditions 50

Natural ways to control hypertension 52
    Change your Diet 52
    DASH Diet.. 54
    Starting DASH diet 56
    Tips on DASH diet.. 57
    Pritikin Diet 58

Exercise 61
    What Type of Exercise Is Best for Hypertension 61
    Specific tips on Exercise with Hypertension. 64
    How Often Should You Exercise 65
    When you should stop exercising 65

Manage your weight.. 67

Alternative ways to reduce high blood pressure 69
    Acupuncture for Hypertension 69
    Natural or Herbal Remedies for Hypertension 71
    Hibiscus Tea for High Blood Pressure 72
    Garlic for Hypertension.. 74

Food supplements for hypertension... 77
    Coenzyme Q10 (CoQ10).. 77
    Omega-3 fatty acids 77

Meditation for Hypertension 79

Simple steps to control your hypertension................................. 81

Conclusion.. 82

Other Books by Dr. Shahriar Mostafa 83
    Diagnosed with Diabetes. Now What!   Smallest Book with Everything You Need to Know 83

Type One Diabetes: Smallest book with everything you need to know 84

Type 2 Diabetes: Smallest book with everything you need to know 85

Pregnancy & Diabetes: Smallest Book with Everything You need to know 86

Notes

The book is designed to save your time searching information on high blood pressure.

Please remember, this book is not a prescription. Do not change, increase, start or skip any ongoing treatment without consulting your doctor. You can use information from this book to ask and consult your doctor for specific treatment.

Every effort has been made to make this book as complete and as accurate as possible. However, there may be mistakes both typographical and in content. The opinion expressed in this book is personal opinion, diagnosis or treatment. You may disagree with the content. The statistical data presented in the book may be changed due to time or newer studies.

Therefore, this text should be used only as a general guide and not as the ultimate source of information.

The information provided here is medical information, learned from medical textbooks and journals and websites. All this information is also available on the Internet. The book is designed to save time searching information.

Healthcare is ever changing, new data is added every year, new treatment emerges. This book will be updated every year. As you have purchased this book, I like to thank you and send you future editions free.

Please send me an email to dr.shahriar@doctor.com with "Hypertension " in the subject line so I can send you future editions of this ebook completely free.

Please post a review of this book if you like or dislike this book. Your review will help people with hypertension to find and get this book. It's an essential book for them. And I thank you in advance for your effort.

Hypertension or High blood pressure.

There is no absolute value in blood pressure, the normal range depends on age, sex, and other factors.

Hypertension is a medical term, it means high blood pressure. The word hypertension seems like it means anxiety, tension or hyperactive personality but it does not indicate that.

Our body is an amazing machine. It's made up of trillions of cells. All these cells need food and oxygen to survive and function. To provide food and oxygen to every cell, we have a very efficient system. It is called the cardiovascular system. The cardiovascular system consists of the heart, blood vessels, and blood. Through our veins and arteries, blood carries and supply all the trillions of cells food and oxygen.

We need a pump to force blood to flow inside vessels, heart works as the pump. The heart is so efficient it pumps 2,000 gallons of blood through 60,000 miles of blood vessels nonstop every day all your life.

This pumping action of the heart creates pressure. So, Blood Pressure (BP) is the force of the blood pushing against the inner walls of your blood vessels as it circulates throughout the body. For many reasons, this pressure may increase from average level. When there is persistently Increased pressure, we call the condition Hypertension or High Blood Pressure.

The blood pressure reading is measured in millimeters of mercury (mmHg) There are two components of blood pressure reading:

When the heart is constricting, or beating the pressure is highest. It is called SYSTOLIC pressure.

And when the heart is relaxing between heartbeats the pressure is at its lowest point called DIASTOLIC pressure.

For example, a blood pressure reading is usually written or mentioned as 120/80 mmHg, or "120 over 80". Here SYSTOLIC pressure is 120 and the DIASTOLIC pressure is 80.

There is no absolute value in blood pressure, the normal range depends on age, sex and other factors. Blood pressure rises with each heartbeat and falls when our heart relaxes between beats. It changes in small level from minute to minute with changes in position, movement, exercise, stress or during sleep.

Usually, when we are referring to normal blood pressure, it's for an adult age 20 or over and it's less than 120 to 110 systolic and less than 80 to 70 diastolic.

So, when do we call a blood pressure as Hypertension? The definition varies worldwide. A standard most of the doctors follow worldwide is given below.

"The Joint National Committee on Prevention, Detection, Evaluation, and Treatment of High Blood Pressure has classified blood pressure measurements into several categories. According to this guideline;

Normal blood pressure is a systolic pressure less than 120 and diastolic pressure less than 80 mm Hg.

"Prehypertension" is a systolic pressure of 120-139 or a diastolic pressure of 80-89 mmHg.

Stage 1 Hypertension is a systolic pressure of 140-159 or a diastolic pressure of 90-99 mmHg.

Stage 2 Hypertension is a systolic pressure of 160 or greater or a diastolic pressure of 100 or higher.

Stage 3 Hypertension is systolic pressure of 180 or higher or diastolic pressure of 110 or greater

In the case of children up to 1 year of age, the normal range is systolic 100 to 75 and diastolic 70 to 50. Children from 1 year to up to 5 years of age normal range is systolic 110 to 80 and diastolic 80 to 50. Children from 1 year to up to 3 years of age normal range is systolic 110 to 85, and diastolic blood pressure is 80 to 50. In teenage average systolic is 120 to 85 and diastolic 80 to 55."

The purpose of this staging is to help doctors to choose the best treatment option for various levels of hypertension.

Risk factors for developing high blood pressure

Risk factors tell you that you have increased chance of becoming hypertensive and you need to start preventive measure as soon as possible

High blood pressure is a common disease of epidemic proportions. It is a global public health issue. For most doctors, it is the single most common chronic disease encountered in practice. It has been estimated that in Western countries somewhere between 15 and 20 percent of the adult population have high blood pressure.

Studies have shown that there are some common factors present in hypertensive patients. These common elements are then named as risk factors.

If present, risk factors tell you that you have increased a chance of becoming hypertensive and you need to start preventive measure as soon as possible.

Family history

Studies have proven genetic factors play a significant role in hypertension. We inherit risk of hypertension from our parents. If your parents or close blood relatives have had hypertension, you are more likely to develop it. You also pass this risk factor onto your children.

That's why it's important for children as well as adults to have regular blood pressure checks if family history of hypertension is present.

You can't control the risk factor you inherit, but you can take steps to prevent hypertension and live a healthy life. Focus on other risk factors (overweight, stress, diet etc.) and work on preventing them.

Through Lifestyle choices, you can prevent hypertension even if you have a strong family history.

Race/Ethnicity

There is a relation in between blood pressure and ethnicity. Studies have proven that "High blood pressure is more common in African American adults than in Caucasian or Hispanic American adults. Compared to other ethnic groups, African Americans Tend to get high blood pressure earlier in life. On average they have higher blood pressure numbers."

You have to double your efforts to control hypertension if you are an African American.

Advanced age

The frightening reality is that most of us will get high blood pressure when we are 60. As we age, we all are at greater risk for high blood pressure and cardiovascular disease.

With aging, blood vessels lose its flexibility and become hard. This hardening causes an increase in blood pressure.

The chance of rupture of blood vessels causing a stroke or heart attack also increases with age.

You need to follow specific steps from an early age to prevent developing hypertension.

Gender-related risk patterns

Gender plays a mixed pattern. Studies have shown, up to 45 years' age-group of women get hypertension more than men, then in the age group 45 to 64 both males and females gets it in similar rate. Again in the age group 64 or more the risk is more in women than men. Overall women tend to develop high blood pressure than men.

If you are a woman, you need to be extra cautious about high blood pressure.

Cause of High Blood Pressure

Unusually for most adults, there's no identifiable cause responsible for high blood pressure.

Your Blood pressure may gradually rise over the years. This type of high blood pressure, without any particular reason, is called primary or essential hypertension.

Don't let the name confuse you, the name doesn't mean this blood pressure is primary and needs no control, nor it is essential for you. It's also not essential to keep at the high level.

On the other hand, some high blood pressure has an underlying identifiable condition or cause. This type of high blood pressure is called secondary hypertension. Because it's secondary to a particular cause.

Usually, secondary hypertension tends to appear suddenly and often show higher blood pressure level than primary hypertension.

We can get secondary Hypertension in following conditions

- Kidney problems
- Adrenal gland tumors
- Thyroid problems
- Certain defects in blood vessels we're born with (congenital)
- Certain medications, such as cold remedies, decongestants, over-the-counter pain relievers and some prescription drugs.
- Illegal drugs, such as cocaine and amphetamines
- Alcohol abuse or chronic alcohol use

There are some other causes responsible for increasing blood pressure. These causes can also be called risk factors because if present they increase the risk of high blood pressure.

Overweight and obesity

This is the single most important cause and a risk factor for high blood pressure. Being overweight increases your chances of developing high blood pressure to a certainty. A body mass index between 25 and 30 is considered overweight. A body mass index over 30 is considered obese.

BMI is a scale to classify obesity. Your weight and height are needed to calculate BMI.

You can easily calculate your body mass index using web apps available online. If the BMI is not in ideal range, you need to manage your weight.

Excess weight increases the strain on the heart. Obesity comes with other conditions. Usually, the level of bad cholesterol (LDL) and triglycerides are high. This condition medically called dyslipidemia increase blood pressure. The bad fats get deposited inside blood vessels and make it narrow and hard causing hypertension.

if you lose as little as 10 to 20 pounds, it can help lower your blood pressure, and that's a start.

Lack of physical activity

Now we work, connect and enjoy more from our desk. Physical activity is ignored. Lack of physical activity causes not only high blood pressure but also many other physical conditions such as obesity, diabetes even depression. Physical activity is good for your heart and circulatory system. A physically inactive lifestyle increases the chance of high blood pressure, heart disease, blood vessel disease and stroke. Inactivity also makes it easier to become overweight or obese. Obesity also is a strong risk factor for high blood pressure.

Diet

healthy food choices can actually lower blood pressure and even prevent it.

Your Diet may cause high blood pressure, and interestingly it can prevent it. Depending on your choice, diet plays a significant role in causing or preventing high blood pressure. Nowadays almost everyone knows that a diet high in salt and fat and low in nutritional value increased the risk for High Blood Pressure and other conditions. And a diet rich in mineral and nutrients with low fat and salt can keep you healthy and prolong your life.

The point is we need to apply this knowledge to our life. We all need good nutrition from a variety of food sources. A diet that's high in calories, fats and sugars and low in essential nutrients also lead to weak heart as well as to obesity leading to hypertension.

Also, salt is another important factor. Some people are "salt sensitive," meaning a high salt (sodium) diet raises their high blood pressure. Salt keeps excess fluid in the body causing increased blood volume. With increased blood volume, your heart has to work more with more force causing a rise in blood pressure.

On the other side, healthy food choices can actually lower blood pressure and prevent it.

Alcohol

Heavy and regular use of alcohol can increase blood pressure dramatically. It can also cause heart failure, stroke, and irregular heartbeats. If you drink, limit your alcohol consumption to no more than two drinks per day for men and one drink per day for women.

Other Possible contributing factors for developing high blood pressure

There is some connection between blood pressure and the following factors, but study has not proven yet that they actually cause high blood pressure.

Stress

We have a common conception that stress and stressful situation causes high blood pressure. It's true that stress and stressful condition temporarily increase blood pressure, but studies have not proven that stress itself can cause long-term high blood pressure.

Some studies show a relationship between coronary heart disease risk and stress in a person's life. Some people under stress eats more and eats a less healthy diet to cope with stressful situations. They may put off physical activity, drink, smoke or misuse drugs. All these results in increased risk of developing hypertension.

Smoking and second-hand smoke

kick the habit as soon as you can.

There is no excuse of smoking. You need to stop, make others quit smoking. Smoking temporarily raises blood pressure causing damaged arteries. So even a single stick is harmful. Secondhand smoke or exposure to other people's smoke increases the risk of heart disease in nonsmokers. You should kick the habit as soon as you can.

Following is an excellent book on quitting cigarette. Take a look if you are a smoker.

The new trend of Vape or vaporized nicotine is still too new to comment. The nicotine in vape is known to raise blood pressure temporarily. Vape needs long term study to be declared safe or unsafe regarding hypertension.

But studies have proven vape or e-cigarettes has a significant role in quitting cigarettes.

You can read the following book to use vape or e-cigarettes to quit tobacco smoking.

Sleep Apnea

This is an unusual cause leading to high blood pressure.

"Some 12 million Americans have sleep apnea", according to National Heart, Lung, and Blood Institute. Sleep Apnea is an unusual but now common sleep disorder in which tissues in the throat collapse and block the airway during sleep. Then brain forces the sleeper awake enough to cough or gulp air and open the trachea. But after a few minutes, the whole cycle starts all over again. This inadequate sleep for a long time causes severe fatigue during the day make it difficult to perform tasks that require alertness. Sleep apnea is a proven risk factor for high blood pressure, heart failure, diabetes and stroke.

Obesity may play a significant role in sleep apnea.

Symptoms of Hypertension

Usually, the only way we find out that we have high blood pressure when it is measured.

It is alarming to know that more than 68 million Americans have hypertension and 33% of them doesn't even know it. The disease is increasingly affecting more and more by almost 15 to 18 million or more every 10 years.

Most of the time there is no symptom of Hypertension. You may have a common misconception that people with hypertension always experience symptoms, but the reality is most hypertensive people have no symptoms at all. Over time severe damage to your arteries, heart, and brain can occur before hypertension is diagnosed. That's why Hypertension is called "Silent Killer."

Hypertension is usually diagnosed by a healthcare professional during a routine checkup.

Sometimes and not in everyone hypertension causes symptoms such as

- Headache,
- Shortness of breath,
- Dizziness,
- Chest pain,
- Palpitations and
- Nose bleeds.

If you have any of these symptoms, Do not ignore them. These symptoms do not confirm that you have hypertension. You may have these symptoms for other diseases. But It is always wise to report symptoms to your doctor as well as to have your blood pressure regularly checked.

If you have risk factors such as obesity, smoking, high cholesterol and family history of hypertension, it is especially important to pay attention to your blood pressure reading.

Increasing age more than 55 years needs regular blood pressure monitoring at least once every 6 months.

Sometimes when blood pressure becomes extremely high, you may have an unusually strong headache, chest pain, difficulty breathing, or difficulty breathing during physical work or exercise. If you have any of these symptoms, consult your doctor for an evaluation as soon as possible.

Diagnosis of Hypertension

Hypertension is usually diagnosed by a healthcare professional during a routine checkup.

Hypertension does not show any obvious symptom unless there are complications such as stroke, heart failure, kidney disease etc. Hypertension is usually diagnosed by a healthcare professional during a routine checkup.

Blood pressure levels are not as stable as cholesterol or body weight but tend to vary in every measurement. Usually during the first visit to the doctor's office blood pressure reading is higher. Also, blood pressure is generally higher in the first measurement than if it's measured 2 or 3 times 10 minutes apart. Good thing this false high blood pressure tends to become regular in following visits.

You can't be diagnosed as hypertensive in one isolated visit. Usually, repeated measurements taken during at least 2 to 3 different visits to the doctor's office is needed to confirm the diagnosis of Hypertension.

The diagnosis of hypertension is made when either

the systolic blood pressure is persistently higher than 140 mmHg

or when the diastolic is greater than 90 mmHg or two conditions coexist.

Sometimes we need to monitor blood pressure for 24 hours before we can be confident about the diagnosis of hypertension.

Problems with uncontrolled hypertension

Every year complications of hypertension such as stroke or heart attack or failure are responsible for more than 9.4 million deaths worldwide.

Hypertension or High blood pressure causes many problems when left untreated. It is one of the leading causes of heart disease and stroke. It also causes kidney disease, a particular type of dementia and eye problems. If we do not take steps to control high blood pressure it affects;

Our brain - High blood pressure is one of the leading causes of stroke. As the pressure is high, blood vessels supplying brain rupture more often causing a stroke. It can also lead to a particular form of dementia called vascular dementia caused by rupture or destruction of tiny vessels supplying the brain.

Our heart and blood vessels - High blood pressure can severely damage your blood vessels. Long term uncontrolled hypertension causes enlargement of the heart. Enlargement of the heart is dangerous, leading to heart failure.

Our kidneys - kidneys have a vital role in removing waste products from our body. High blood pressure can damage kidneys by damaging its filtering structure and vessels. The problem is, damage to our kidneys also raises blood pressure. This is a dangerous cycle. When uncontrolled this leads to complete failure of kidneys.

Our eyes and limbs - High blood pressure does not just affect internal organs. It also damages the blood vessels throughout the body such as eyes and limbs, causing loss or decreased sight and mobility problems.

Studies show your risk for stroke or heart attack double with only 10 mmHg rise in blood pressure. So even a small increase is dangerous.

Every year complications of hypertension such as stroke or heart attack or failure are responsible for more than 9.4 million deaths worldwide. Individually Hypertension causes half of the deaths (51%) due to stroke and almost half (45%) the deaths attributable to heart failure.

It's crucial that you control your high blood pressure and keep it controlled lifelong for a healthy and long life.

Treatment Options for High Blood Pressure

You may need to continue treatment for Hypertension the rest of your life, even if your blood pressure becomes normal.

Hypertension is a chronic disease, it means you have to be prepared to continue treatment for a long time. Sometimes you may need to continue treatment the rest of your life, even if your blood pressure becomes normal.

As your diagnosis is confirmed as hypertension, you face a common confusion of Choosing the right treatment plan

If you know some general information about the treatment options available, you can discuss your thoughts or plans with your doctor. Keep in mind your doctor is the best person to advise your treatment but it's you who will decide the treatment plan. With information, you can take a correct and informed decision.

General Treatment Guideline for High Blood Pressure

Treatment to control high blood pressure is individualized. Sometimes you may need to go through trial and error under the supervision of your doctor to choose the medicine and dose right for you.

Treatment of hypertension depends on multiple factors. Most of the time the treatment to control high blood pressure is individualized. Sometimes you may need to go through trial and error under the supervision of your doctor to choose the medicine and dose right for you. Your doctor plays a significant role in selecting the best treatment. Treatment also depends on the type of hypertension you have.

Following are treatment guidelines used by doctors worldwide to treat hypertension

Prehypertension
Treatment with drugs or medicines is not necessary for prehypertension stage.

American Guidelines for Hypertension (JNC-7, 2003) use the term prehypertension. In pre-hypertension, the systolic reading is within 120 mmHg to 139 mmHg, or the diastolic reading is within 80 mmHg to 89 mmHg. Or both systolic and diastolic can be high.

Prehypertension is a warning sign that you may get high blood pressure soon. The term prehypertension is used to create early awareness. According to the American Heart Association, "59 million people in the U.S. have prehypertension".

But on the other hand, European Society of Hypertension, British Society of Hypertension and Hellenic Society for The Study of Hypertension do not use the term or classification of Prehypertension.

According to those guidelines, a systolic pressure between 120 mmHg to 129 mmHg or the diastolic pressure between 80 mmHg to 84 mmHg is the standard range of blood pressure. According to these guidelines Systolic pressure 130 to 139 mmHg or diastolic 85 to 89 mmHg, or both are termed as High normal blood pressure.

People with prehypertension or High normal blood pressure have a greater risk of other cardiovascular diseases such as stroke. Most of the time risk factors for hypertension such as high cholesterol, obesity, and diabetes are seen more in people with prehypertension than in those with normal blood pressure.

The goal of Prehypertension is to start lifestyle changes early for the prevention of hypertension. Prehypertension needs monitoring of blood pressure regularly, so it allows prompt treatment if blood pressure becomes higher.

Treatment with drugs or medicines is not necessary for prehypertension stage.

Here are some strategies to help you manage prehypertension:

- Lose weight if you are overweight. Obese people has a risk of developing prehypertension 20% more. On the other hand, even a modest amount of weight loss reduces the risk.
- Exercise regularly. Exercise helps you lose weight. Exercise also helps lower blood pressure.
- Eat plenty of fruits, vegetables, whole grains, fish, and low-fat dairy. A specific diet plan such as DASH can prevent hypertension as well as lower blood pressure.
- Reduce salt/sodium in your diet. You should take less than 2,300 milligrams of sodium per day (2300 mg is about 1 teaspoon of table salt).

- It's important to get your blood pressure checked regularly. You can monitor your blood pressure between doctor's visits with a home blood pressure monitor.

Stage 1 Hypertension

At stage 1 hypertension start with lifestyle modification, there is a strong possibility that you will not need any drugs to control stage 1 hypertension

If your systolic blood pressure is between 140 and 159 or your diastolic pressure between 90 and 99, you are considered to be in hypertension stage 1. Stage 1 hypertension occurs more frequently in older individuals (age 65 and more), women and African Americans.

Untreated stage 1 hypertension leads to atherosclerosis. In atherosclerosis, arteries became hard and lost its elasticity with increased risk of stroke, heart attack and kidney disease. In stage 1 hypertension your heart needs to work harder to pump the blood inside the body.

At stage 1 hypertension start with lifestyle modification, there is a strong possibility that you will not need any drugs to control stage 1 hypertension. But some of us will need to take medicine to control blood pressure even on stage 1. The JNC 7 report recommends that "the first medication to use is a thiazide-type diuretic." A diuretic is a drug that lowers blood pressure by helping your body get rid of extra fluid. Diuretics are usually very effective, have fewer side effects, and are inexpensive. Diuretics are used not only to reduce blood pressure but also to decrease the risk of heart disease and stroke.

If you are African-American risk for complications of hypertension is higher. So the current guideline is that African-Americans with blood pressure 145mm Hg or more should start with a combined blood pressure medicine.

Stage 2 Hypertension

If you have Stage 2 Hypertension, you must consult your doctor and start immediate treatment.

According to current guidelines, Systolic blood pressure is 160 mm Hg or higher or diastolic 100 mm Hg or greater is called stage 2 hypertension. Stage 2 hypertension is also known as late high blood pressure or severe high blood pressure.

Stage 2 hypertension is a dangerous form of high blood pressure. It needs more frequent blood pressure checks and more careful monitoring.

If you have Stage 2 Hypertension, you must consult your doctor and start immediate treatment. Initially, you have to start lifestyle changes, including:

- Quit smoking.
- Maintain a healthy weight.
- Consume a diet rich in fruits, vegetables, and low-fat dairy products.
- Limit salt in your diet.
- Limit alcohol intake.
- Exercise at least 30 minutes per day. Simple aerobic exercise such as walking, jogging, strength training, yoga or cardio workout like cycling.

In stage 2 hypertension it's a strong possibility that in addition to lifestyle changes you will need medicine preferably a two-drug therapy. It will be advised by your doctor. Following drugs are usually used to treat Stage 2 hypertension:

- ACE inhibitors – they allow blood vessels to widen by preventing angiotensin (a hormone) from forming.
- Angiotensin II receptor blockers - by blocking the action of angiotensin these drugs allow blood vessels to relax.
- Beta blockers - block particular nerve and hormone signals to your heart and blood vessels causing relaxed heart and blood vessel leading to lower blood pressure.
- Calcium channel blockers - prevent calcium ions from going into heart muscle and blood vessel muscle causing a widening of blood vessels leading to lower blood pressure.
- Renin inhibitors - slow down the production of renin, which is an enzyme produced by your kidneys that increase blood pressure. Without renin, your blood pressure lowers to an average level.

Stage 3 Hypertension

Stage 3 hypertension is a medical emergency

Stage 3 is an incredibly high blood pressure. In stage 3 pressure becomes more than 180/110 mmHg. It is also called severe hypertension. Stage 3 hypertension needs urgent medical treatment with close monitoring.

Remember, stage 3 hypertension is a medical emergency and may require treatment in a hospital setting.

Medicines used in Hypertension

An important aspect of hypertension medications is the prevention of complication. Most of the time medicine is given to keep the cardiovascular system (Heart, blood vessels) healthy and to stop the damage.

The most concern about every medicine we take is the side effect. As drugs of hypertension need to be taken a long time sometimes all your life we worry about the side effects more. Is it possible to avoid drugs entirely? The answer is complicated. Control of high blood pressure needs multiple factors. It is proven that lifestyle modification and modifying your diet can control high blood pressure. But to control stage 2 and stage 3 hypertension medicine is essential.

Another important aspect of hypertension drugs is the prevention of complication. Most of the time medicine is given to keep the cardiovascular system (Heart, blood vessels) healthy and to stop the damage. They prevent premature aging of the cardiovascular system. In reality, the primary goal of hypertension medicine is to avoid, not to control blood pressure.

We have many kinds of hypertension medicine working on different mechanisms to control blood pressure. Hypertension treatment with drugs is different from other treatment. Blood pressure medicine needs individual adjustment of dose. The choice of drug is also individualized. Initially, you may have to go through a trial and error phase to find the right drug and perfect dose. Don't be alarmed if your doctor frequently changes your drug or dose initially. We take several factors to choose the antihypertensive medicine. Such as

- Your general health
- Sex
- Age
- Severity of the high blood pressure;
- Any additional, underlying medical condition
- Potential side effects

If you have Bronchial asthma, heart disease, diabetes or gout. In these conditions, certain drugs are especially good, but others may be contraindicated.

The medicine on which you will respond depends on factors such as:

- The causes of your high blood pressure.
- How high your blood pressure is.
- How your body responds to different high blood pressure medicines.
- Any other health problems such as diabetes or high cholesterol you might have.

Most drugs for lowering high blood pressure are effective up to 24 hours so, most of the time one tablet is taken in the morning or night is enough to control high blood pressure. But when high blood pressure is severe or resistant to treatment, more than one tablet may be needed. Some of us may need three or more drugs to control blood pressure. There is evidence that low doses of two blood pressure lowering drugs are more effective than either given alone. Moreover, low dose of two drugs causes less side effect.

There may be some trial and error testing to find the combination of high blood pressure medicine that works best for you.

Many people need more than one type of high blood pressure medication to get the best results. Your doctor will decide which one is best for you. Choosing the best medicine may need some trial and error, do not be alarmed if initially, your doctor changes drug or dose too often.

You need to have a treatment goal if you are taking or consider taking medicines for Hypertension. The treatment goal depends on your age, health status and if you have another disease such as diabetes.

- As a general rule 120 /8,0 mm Hg or lower is the recommended blood pressure goal.
- If you are a healthy adult with age 60 or more, your goal should be Less than150/90 mm Hg.
- Less than140/90 mm Hg is recommended If you're a healthy adult younger than age 60
- If you have chronic kidney disease, diabetes or coronary artery disease or are at high risk of coronary artery disease your goal should be Less than140/90 mm Hg.

We always worry about taking any medicine for their side effects. As we have to take hypertension drugs for a long time considering the safety of the drug is crucial. But you need not worry. Medicines treating high blood pressure is extensively tested for their safety in long time use. In reality, not taking drugs may harm you more than the mild side effects. The side effects depend upon the particular drug given, dose, and other factors.

Although antihypertensive drugs are generally well tolerated, still they have some side effects;

Some of the time when starting High blood pressure medicines for the first time, it may lower blood pressure abruptly. This sudden low blood pressure may cause dizziness, drowsiness, lightheadedness, or feeling of fainting with sudden movement. These symptoms usually subside after a few weeks.

Following are the common medicines used to treat high blood pressure along with information on their safety and side effects.

Diuretics

If you need medicine for hypertension diuretics are used as a first choice. Diuretics are a class of drugs. They work on the kidneys and wash out more salt and water from the body. Removing water results in less blood volume circulating in your blood vessels. Less volume means heart works less with less force, leading to lower blood pressure. Diuretics remove water from your body through urine, so there is an increase in frequency and volume of urine. That's why they are called "water pills."

There are many drugs in the class diuretics. For hypertension, most used one is thiazide diuretics.

Sometimes you may need a combination of two diuretics to control hypertension. Some examples of combination diuretics are:

Spironolactone and Hydrochlorothiazide

Hydrochlorothiazide and Triamterene

Amiloride Hydrochloride and Hydrochlorothiazide

Usually, for most of the people, there is no side effect of hypertension medicine. A few of us may have mild side effects. The side effects usually occur when trying a new drug or increased dose. Most of the time these side effects subside over time. If you feel the side effects for a long time, then you may need to change the drug.

Possible side-effects of -diuretic include:

- An increased need to go to the toilet (Increased Urine)
- Feeling thirsty
- Feeling dizzy, weak, lethargic or sick
- Low blood pressure when moving from lying or sitting to standing
- Muscle cramps
- Skin rash
- Increase Complications of Gout due to increased uric acid levels
- Increased blood glucose levels
- Erectile Dysfunction in men.

The important side effect of Diuretics is it may lower the amount of potassium in your body. Low potassium in the blood is termed as hypokalemia. It is a dangerous condition. Your doctor will monitor your potassium level in blood from time to time.

Things you need to be careful when taking diuretics are;

- You should take your diuretic in the morning as they produce more urine than normal. This will help you avoid having to get up in the night to go to the toilet frequently.
- You need to have regular blood and urine tests to check potassium and blood sugar levels.

- Thiazide diuretic with a beta-blocker increase risk of developing diabetes. Make sure you are not taking them together.

Check with your doctor before taking any other medicines, including over the counter drugs.

Beta-Blockers

Beta blockers are a group of drug work by blocking the effects of the hormone epinephrine, also known as adrenaline. This hormone (epinephrine/ adrenaline) increases heart rate and constrict blood vessels. When you take beta blockers the action of the hormone is blocked, your heart beats more slowly and with less force, thereby reducing blood pressure. Beta blockers also help blood vessels to relax, which improve blood flow.

Beta blockers are not the first choice for treating hypertension. If other drugs as diuretics could not control your hypertension Beta blockers are used. Most of the time Beta blocker is used in combination with two or more drugs. The combination may include angiotensin-converting enzyme (ACE) inhibitors, diuretics or calcium channel blockers.

Beta blocked is relatively safe for long-term use. Some side effects happen with Beta blocker which is mild and does not carry a risk to your health.

Common side effects of beta blockers include:

- Fatigue
- Cold hands or feet
- Weight gain
- Less common side effects include:
- Shortness of breath
- Trouble sleeping

- Depression

Generally, Beta blockers are not used in people with asthma because it can trigger severe asthma attacks. In individuals who have diabetes, beta-blockers may hide signs of low blood sugar, such as rapid heartbeat. You need to monitor your blood sugar regularly while on Beta blocker. Beta blockers can slightly increase triglyceride level in blood. And a modest decrease may occur in HDL (high-density lipoprotein) which is the good cholesterol.

Beta blockers may not work effectively for black and older people, especially when taken without other blood pressure medications.

You shouldn't abruptly stop taking a beta-blocker because doing so could increase your risk of a heart attack or other heart problems. When taking beta blockers, you should

Beta blocker lowers the heart rate. You need to learn to check your pulse. Check your pulse regularly to make sure your heart rate is not too slow (less than 60).

Beta blockers sometimes cause higher blood sugar levels. On the other hand, beta-blockers can hide your symptoms of low blood sugar. You need to be alert if you are a diabetic taking beta blockers.

Alpha-blockers for Hypertension

Blood vessels of our body have a muscle layer responsible for regulation of blood flow. There is receptor present in all the muscles. These receptors work like buttons, when they are activated, muscles tighten leading to tightening of blood vessels. Then heart has to work hard with more force causing high blood pressure.

Alpha blockers block these specific receptors so receptors can't be activated leading to lower blood pressure.

Alpha-blockers are usually the third or fourth choice to control blood pressure. Because alpha blockers can only lower blood pressure, they don't have protective ability to protect and prevent heart attack or stroke, like other blood pressure medicine. Most of the time alpha blocker is used in combination with two or more drugs.

If you are starting Alpha Blocker for the first time you need to take the first dose at bedtime. Alpha Blocker causes a marked low blood pressure initially so you may experience dizziness and feeling of fainting or may faint when moving suddenly (e.g. suddenly standing from the toilet). This effect is called first dose effect and will subside after some time. So initially take Alpha Blocker before going to bed.

Other side effects of alpha blocker include:

- Headache
- Pounding heartbeat
- Weakness
- Dizziness
- Weight gain
- Sudden drops in blood pressure when -sitting up or standing up
- Swollen legs or ankles
- Tremor
- Rash or itchiness of the skin
- Problems with erections in men.

Alpha blockers can increase or decrease the effects of other medications Such as beta blockers, calcium channel blockers or drugs for erectile dysfunction. Before taking an alpha blocker, remember to inform your doctor if you are taking other medicines.

Alpha blocker is avoided in women because they can cause stress incontinence and loss of bladder control. If you are pregnant, breastfeeding or planning a pregnancy, do not take alpha blockers. Alpha Blocker is avoided in patients with heart failure, liver disease or decreased kidney function. Alpha Blocker is not given Parkinson's' disease.

ACE inhibitors

Normal blood pressure is regulated in our body by some mechanism. One of these mechanisms is by a hormone called Angiotensin. Angiotensin tightens blood vessel and increases pressure. Angiotensin Converting Enzyme (ACE) inhibitors are a class of high blood pressure medicine which prevents our body from making angiotensin II from Angiotensin.

Angiotensin-converting enzyme (ACE) inhibitors relax or open up the blood vessels to improve circulation blood and lower blood pressure. ACE inhibitors also decrease the amount of work your heart has to do.

ACE inhibitor drugs are given as a first choice if you need medicine to control your blood pressure. They are the drug of choice for young people (less than 55 years of age) who developed hypertension.

Like any drug, ACE inhibitors have some side effects. They may include:

- Cough. Some people not in everyone ACE inhibitors cause a persistent dry cough. If you get it then you have to stop this class of drugs.
- ACE inhibitors may cause red, itchy skin or rash.
- The sudden change of postures like standing from sitting position you may feel dizziness, lightheadedness or fainting. It is due to sudden fall in blood pressure.
- A salty & metallic taste or a reduced ability to taste.

You may experience some physical symptoms such as a sore throat, mouth sores, fast or irregular heartbeat, chest pain, and swelling of feet, ankles and lower legs. It can also cause Swelling of your neck, face, and tongue. You need to consult your doctor immediately if you experience these symptoms. These symptoms may represent a serious emergency.

ACE inhibitors can cause high potassium levels in the blood called as hyperkalemia. This is a potentially life-threatening complication. You should regularly check your potassium level in blood.

High potassium in blood or Hyperkalemia is a dangerous condition, there are some symptoms associated with high potassium such as irregular heartbeat, tingling, and numbness in hand, foot or around lips. It may cause confusion, drowsiness and breathing problem. Be alert for these symptoms. Seek immediate potassium level check and treatment if the symptoms show up.

Some Guidelines for Taking ACE Inhibitors

- Always take ACE inhibitors on an empty stomach one hour before meals.
- Monitor your blood pressure and kidney functions regularly when on ACE Inhibitor.
- Salt substitute contains high potassium so do not use salt substitutes while taking ACE Inhibitors. You need to read food labels to choose low-sodium and low-potassium foods.
- You cannot take ACE inhibitors during pregnancy. They can cause death or deformity in the newborn
- ACE inhibitor can pass through breast milk so avoid it if you breastfeed your baby.

Calcium Channel Blockers

Another class of drug used to control blood pressure is called Calcium Channel Blockers (CCB). For the pumping action heart, muscles need calcium ions. CCB blocks the pathway of calcium ions. So, heart muscle gets calcium slowly. The heart stays relaxed. CCB also widens blood vessels, so the heart has to work less all these helps to lower blood pressure to normal level.

Possible side-effects of calcium-channel blockers include:

- Swollen ankles
- Ankle or foot pain
- Constipation
- Skin rashes
- A flushed face
- Headaches
- Dizziness or tiredness
- Swollen or bleeding gums (rarely)

If you are taking a calcium-channel blocker, you should not drink grapefruit juice. Grapefruit juice makes absorption of CCB rapidly and more. With more drug in your blood cause blood pressure to drop suddenly and dangerously low level.

Calcium Channel Blockers are not used If there is kidney or liver disease along with hypertension.

Angiotensin II Receptor Blockers (ARB)

As I have mentioned earlier, a hormone called Angiotensin helps regulate blood pressure. Angiotensin binds with receptors present in blood vessels and tightens them. Angiotensin Receptor Blockers (ARB) block these receptor keeping the blood vessels relaxed with smooth blood flow, in effect blood pressure lowers to a normal level.

ARB is the first choice if you need two or more combined blood pressure medicine. For younger patients (age less than 55 years), diabetic patients and patients with kidney disease ARB is the drug of choice. ARB has a protective role on kidneys.

If you are pregnant, breastfeeding or planning a pregnancy, you should not be given an angiotensin receptor blocker. Because angiotensin II receptor blockers can injure a developing fetus.

Very few people have side effects with ARB. Possible side effects include:

- Dizziness
- Increased potassium level in blood (hyperkalemia)
- Swelling of tissues (angioedema)
- Diarrhea
- Gross weight loss

Direct Vasodilators

This class of high blood pressure medicine works on blood vessels directly. They relax the muscles in your blood vessel walls. This makes the blood vessels to widen, and blood flows through them more easily. This results in lower blood pressure.

Usually, these drugs are used in resistant hypertension when three or more drugs are needed to control blood pressure. They are also applied in a hypertensive emergency.

Usually, direct vasodilator is used in combination with a diuretic and a beta blocker.

Direct vasodilators have some side effect such as rapid heartbeat, headaches and joint pain.

Central Agonists

Our body has amazing mechanisms to maintain our blood pressure in normal level. One of the mechanism maintains blood pressure by increasing or decreasing heart rate using signals from our brain. Centrally acting drugs binds to the receptor present in our brain and activate them. Active receptors send a signal to the heart to slow down. Lower heart rate decreases the blood pressure. It also causes to relax our blood vessels.

Due to strong side effects, these drugs are usually not used. Side effects include:

- Fatigue
- Drowsiness or sedation
- Dizziness
- Impotence
- Constipation
- Abnormally slow heart rate
- Dry mouth
- Headache
- Fever

If you are taking Central Agonist never stop the drug suddenly. When central agonists have stopped abruptly, it causes a sudden and very high rise in blood pressure, which is very dangerous.

Direct Renin Inhibitors

Direct Renin Inhibitors are new drugs for hypertension. How does it work! You may be surprised to know that normal blood pressure level is maintained by our kidneys. Kidneys produce an enzyme called "Renin" which has an active role in regulating blood pressure. Direct renin inhibitors block renin to work. Without the trigger event of renin, our blood vessels stay relaxed and wide. Blood flows smoothly causing blood pressure to decrease.

Tekturna is a direct renin inhibitor. As high blood pressure medicine, Tekturna has used alone or in combination other medicines.

As direct renin inhibitors are a new type of medicine for high blood pressure. Studies are ongoing to know about the safety of the drug after prolonged use.

Take direct renin inhibitors only if prescribed by your doctor.

Peripheral-Acting Adrenergic Blockers

Peripheral adrenergic blockers as the name imply blocks nerve impulse. By this blocking muscles in our blood vessels relaxes. Less force than needed by heart to keep blood flowing. In turn, the blood pressure decreases.

These medicines are usually not used. If other medicines including combined medicines fail to control blood pressure, then these drugs are used.

Medicine for Specific Conditions

Some specific conditions need specific blood pressure medicine. These recommended medicines have been proved by extensive studies showing more benefit than other drugs. For example;

Diabetic patients with hypertension response more with Angiotensin Converting Enzyme (ACE) Inhibitor. Besides controlling blood pressure ACE inhibitors protects kidney and heart especially in diabetic patients.

The drug class Beta blockers work best for people with heart failure and heart attack. They prevent heart attack besides controlling blood pressure.

Along with lowering high blood pressure Calcium Channel Blockers control symptoms in people with angina caused by inadequate blood supply to heart muscles due to coronary artery disease.

Also, some antihypertensive drugs should not be used in certain conditions. Such as;

ACE inhibitors and angiotensin II receptor blockers (ARBs) must be avoided during pregnancy and breastfeeding.

Gout patients should not get the drugs classified as diuretics or water pills. They can worsen gout.

Combination of medicine

Combination drug therapy — Sometimes and in some people lifestyle modification along with a single medicine could not control blood pressure. Then a combination of two or more drugs used together. Treating high blood pressure needs individualized drug and dose adjustment. So if you're given a combination of medicines don't be worried it's a recommended treatment protocol.

Sometimes If a person has very high blood pressure (e.g., 160/100 mmHg or higher), then combination therapy with two or more drugs can be started from the very beginning of treatment.

The beneficial side of combination therapy are

- They may be more efficient than increasing the dose of the single drug
- Amazingly a combination of medicines has less side effect than a single drug with higher doses.

Natural ways to control hypertension

Lifestyle change can control your blood pressure dramatically without any medicine.

Every drug has some side effect, so initially you should start with lifestyle modification. Lifestyle change can control your blood pressure dramatically without any medicine. As it is the Natural way to control blood pressure it is best for you in ling term. There are lots of studies to prove that lifestyle modification can control and even prevent high blood pressure.

By lifestyle change we grossly mean modification of your diet, some exercise, stop smoking and limiting your alcoholic beverages. There is a strong possibility that you wouldn't need to take any medicine to keep high blood pressure in control if you properly modify your lifestyle.

Change your Diet

Diet is used as a treatment for high blood pressure. Modification of your diet may control your blood pressure without any medicine. On the other hand, you may be at an increased risk of getting high blood pressure if you eat a diet that's low in fiber, high in fat and salt, drink alcohol to excess and smoke.

A healthy diet not only help controlling high blood pressure, but it can also prevent it.

As a general rule, you should eat plenty of

- Fruits
- Vegetables
- Whole grains
- Fish
- Low-fat dairy
- Low in sodium

Your diet should be

- High in potassium
- Magnesium
- Calcium
- Protein
- Fiber.

Avoid foods high in saturated fat such as meats and high-fat dairy. Control trans fat such some margarine, snack foods, and pastries in your diet. Limit high cholesterol containing foods such as organ meats, high-fat dairy, and egg yolks. Eat foods low in saturated and trans-fat and cholesterol, read food labels to choose.

Eat plant-based or vegetarian diet at least 2 days every week. You can add high-protein soy foods to your diet. Increase fruits and vegetables.

Salt keeps excess fluid in the body causing heart to work more. That is a burden on the heart. You must limit salt in your diet. Studies have proven that "A low-sodium diet can lower high blood pressure." According to the recommendation, you should aim for less than 2,300 milligrams of sodium (salt) daily which is about 1 teaspoon of table salt.

Drinking excess alcohol increase blood pressure. Limit drinking.

DASH Diet

DASH stands for Dietary Approaches to Stop Hypertension

The DASH diet is a specific diet for patients with High Blood Pressure. It is proven in many studies and highly recommended to control your blood pressure. If you don't want to take medicine for your high blood pressure and plan to manage it naturally, then this particular diet is the answer.

DASH stands for Dietary Approaches to Stop Hypertension. In research studies, people who were on the DASH diet lowered their blood pressure within 2 weeks. Some extensive studies found the following health benefits of the DASH diet.

"DASH (Dietary Approaches to Stop Hypertension Trial): This trial included 459 adults, some with and without diagnosed high blood pressure, and compared three diets including 3,000 mg daily sodium.

- Result - Participants on the DASH diet had the greatest effect of lowering their high blood pressure. The DASH diet lowers blood pressure and LDL (bad) cholesterol compared with a typical American diet alone or a typical American diet with more fruits and vegetables.

DASH-Sodium (DASH Diet, Sodium Intake, and Blood Pressure Trial): This trial randomly assigned 412 participants to a typical American diet or the DASH diet. While on their assigned diet, participants were followed for a month at a high daily sodium level (3,300 mg) and two lower daily sodium levels (2,300 mg and 1,500 mg).

- Result - Blood pressure decreased with each reduction of sodium. The DASH-Sodium diet lowers blood pressure better than a typical American diet at three daily sodium levels. Combining the DASH diet with sodium reduction gives greater health benefits than the DASH diet alone.

The PREMIER clinical trial: The PREMIER trial included 810 participants who were placed into three groups to lower blood pressure, lose weight, and improve health. After 6 months, blood pressure levels declined in all three groups.

- Result - Participants in the established treatment plan who followed the DASH diet had the greatest improvement in their blood pressure. People can lose weight and lower their blood pressure by following the DASH eating plan and increasing their physical activity".

The DASH diet is simple:

- Eat more fruits, vegetables, and low-fat dairy foods
- Avoid foods that are high in saturated fat, cholesterol, and trans fats
- Eat more whole-grain foods, fish, poultry, and nuts
- Limit sodium, sweets, sugary drinks, and red meats

DASH-Sodium – is a modified DASH diet cutting back salt (sodium) to 1,500 milligrams a day. 1500 mg salt is about two-third (2/3) of a teaspoon. This amount includes all sodium taken per day. Including sodium in food products, used in cooking and taken at the table.

Starting DASH diet

The DASH diet is based on a certain number of servings daily from various food groups. Depending on the calorie requirement the number of serving is estimated. It is individualized and usually calculated by a dietitian. But you may calculate your calorie need. And adjusts your diet according to DASH plan.

The DASH diet is calculated with serving. When you're trying to follow DASH diet, you need to know the volume of a particular kind of food is considered a "serving." One serving is:

- 1/2 cup cooked rice or pasta is considered a "serving."
- 1 slice bread is considered a "serving."
- 1 cup raw vegetables or fruit is considered a "serving."
- 1/2 cup cooked veggies or fruit is considered a "serving."
- 8 ounces of milk is considered a "serving."
- 1 teaspoon of olive oil (or any other oil) is considered a "serving."
- 3 ounces of cooked meat is considered a "serving."
- 3 ounces of tofu is considered a "serving."

Following is a sample daily and weekly DASH Eating Plan to give you an idea of the diet. This sample plan a sets goal for a 2,000 Calorie per day:

- Grains: 7-8 servings daily
- Vegetables: 4-5 servings daily
- Fruits: 4-5 servings daily
- Fat-free or Low-fat dairy products: 2-3 servings daily
- Meat, poultry, and fish: less than 2 daily servings
- Nuts, seeds, and dry beans: weekly 4-5 servings
- Fats and oils: less than 3 servings daily
- Sweets: try to limit to less than 5 servings per week.

You need specific changes in the DASH diet if you have other associated conditions such as Diabetes or high cholesterol.

For DASH-Sodium diet - You can limit your salt intake gradually. Start by limiting to 2,400 milligrams of salt (sodium) per day. It's about 1 teaspoon of table salt. Then, once you have adjusted to the low salt diet, cut back to 1,500 milligrams of salt (sodium) per day which is about 2/3 of a teaspoon. These amounts include all sodium eaten, including sodium in food products as well as in what you cook with or add at the table.

Tips on DASH diet

Following are some tips you can use when on DASH or DASH-Sodium diet:

Always add a serving of vegetables at lunch and at dinner.

Add a serving of fruit to your meals or as a snack. Canned and dried fruits are easy to use, but make sure by reading the label that they don't have added sugar or salt.

Use low-fat or fat-free and only half your typical serving of butter, margarine, or salad dressing.

Drink low-fat or skim dairy products instead of full-fat or full cream.

Limit meat to 6 ounces a day. Make some meals vegetarian.

Add more vegetables and beans to your diet.

Unsalted pretzels or nuts, raisins, low-fat or fat-free yogurt, unsalted popcorn without butter or oil, and raw vegetables is a good snacking choice.

You should always read food labels to choose products that are low in salt and fat.

Every individual is different. Our food choices are different so you should consult a dietitian to get an accurate DASH diet plan tailored according to your need and food habit.

Pritikin Diet

There is another Popular diet plan available for high blood pressure called Pritikin diet. The Pritikin Principle or diet is a low-fat diet based on vegetables, grains, and fruits. Nathan Pritikin invented the plan. Robert Pritikin improved the diet. Plant-based foods with very little fat are mainly used in Pritikin diet. The latest Pritikin diet focuses on a most recent concept called calorie density solution.

With calorie density, the concern is not calories in various food but rather how dense they are in any given food. The idea is to choose foods that are not "calorie dense," meaning they have relatively low calories per pound. For example, a pound of raw broccoli has 130 calories (without butter), and a pound of chocolate chip cookies has 2,140 calories.

How the Pritikin Principle Works

Pritikin diet suggests we eat whole, unprocessed, and natural carbohydrate-rich foods, such as grains, vegetables, and fruit. Preferred foods include:

- Brown rice
- Millet
- Barley
- Oats
- Dark green, leafy vegetables
- Onions

- Potatoes
- Squash
- Beans (black turtle beans, chickpeas, lentils, lima and pinto beans)
- Apples
- Pears
- Strawberries
- Bananas

Some processed whole-grain foods, such as oatmeal, white-flour pasta can be included in your diet, as long as you eat it with vegetables.

Other guidelines in Pritikin diet are:

- You can eat small servings of lean beef, chicken, and low-fat dairy products.
- Including fish in your diet is encouraged. Pritikin diet suggests at least three servings of fish per week of salmon or other fish rich in omega-3 fatty acids.
- You have to avoid fried foods, dressing with fat, and fatty sauces.
- Eat three meals a day plus two snacks.
- Avoid salty foods.
- Artificial sweeteners can be used in Pritikin diet.

The Pritikin program gives dramatic results. Blood pressure starts to falls quickly. Studies on the Pritikin Program have shown that this diet reduces the need for blood pressure medicine in many people. One study with 1117 high blood pressure patients demonstrated that on average with Pritikin diet blood pressure is reduced 9% or more. 45% of the patients lowered their high blood pressure medicine and astounding 55% stopped high blood pressure medicine achieving normal range of blood pressure.

You can choose to try both diets (DASH or PRITIKIN) alternatively to see which one works better for you.

Exercise

Regular exercise reduces blood pressure by an average of 6-7 mmHg

Due to urban life and development of technology such as (TV, Computer and mobiles) we have developed a physically inactive lifestyle. Most of our time is spent in sitting or lying using computer, games or mobile, even in the office. This leads to risk factors. Physical inactivity is a major risk factor for developing high blood pressure and the risk increases with age.

Exercise can make a big difference in the prevention of hypertension. And if your blood pressure is already high, exercise can help you control it. Scientific studies have shown that "regular exercise reduces blood pressure by an average of 6-7 mmHg". That's as good as some blood pressure medications.

For some of the hypertensive patients, exercise is enough to reduce blood pressure. There is no need for any blood pressure medication. During exercise, your blood pressure may become a bit high but the pressure becomes low afterward. Studies have shown the effect of only 30 minutes of exercise has an immediate blood pressure lowering effect lasting minutes to hours.

What Type of Exercise Is Best for Hypertension
There are three basic types of exercise:

Easy aerobic exercise such as walking, jogging, jumping rope, bicycling (stationary or outdoor), cross-country skiing, skating, rowing, high- or low-impact aerobics and swimming. Aerobic exercise works best in lowering your blood pressure and make your heart stronger.

Walking is one of the most effective exercises for all levels of high blood pressure and for every age group. Walking gives the best result.

Strength training builds strong muscles that help you burn more calories throughout the day. It's also good for your joints and bones.

Stretching makes you more flexible, helps you move better, and helps prevent injury.

So how does exercise work? Regular physical activity or exercise makes your heart stronger. A stronger heart can pump more blood with less effort. If your heart can work less (low heartbeat) to pump, the force on your arteries decreases, lowering your blood pressure. Also during exercise, there is a temporary increase in your heart rate along with blood pressure, it has a cleansing effect on your blood vessels removing plaques blocking it.

The exact duration and type of exercise for blood pressure management is not necessary. However, the current guidelines listed by the American College of Sports Medicine recommend "you should start with 30 minutes of moderate aerobic exercise in the form of walking, running or cycling at least five days per week. Regular physical activity at least 30 minutes most days of the week can lower your blood pressure by 4 to 9 millimeters of mercury (mm Hg). Remember that you need to be consistent in your workout if you stop regular exercising, your blood pressure becomes high again.

Research has found that too much sedentary time can contribute to many health conditions including high blood pressure. If in your workplace, you have to sit for long hours every day, try to break the amount of time into hourly chunks. Do any physical activity for 5 minutes, you may get up to get a drink of water or walk a little inside the office or climb some stairs every hour. Consider setting a reminder in your to-do list, calendar or on your smartphone. Following are some tips to help you;

- Exercise at the same time every day. It will become a regular part of your routine, and it will be harder to skip.
- Wear comfortable clothes when you work out.
- It's best to take your blood pressure before and after you exercise.
- Set realistic goals for yourself that you think you can achieve.
- Find an exercise "buddy." This will help you stay motivated and enjoy it more.

Most people with high blood pressure can exercise safely. But as exercise makes your heart work harder, you need to be careful, especially if you're just starting or your blood pressure is moderately or very high. If your blood pressure is moderately high (stage 2 hypertension), you may need to take medicine to reach a lower level of blood pressure before you may start exercising. If your blood pressure is very high (stage 3 hypertension), you should not start any new activity without consulting your doctor. In general;

- If your Blood pressure level is below 90/60 or lower then you have low blood pressure, It may lead to dizziness even fainting, speak to your doctor or nurse before starting any new exercise with low blood pressure.
- If Blood pressure in the range of 90/60-140/90 It is safe to exercise and be more active.

- If your Blood pressure in range of 140/90 – 179/99. Exercising with moderate intensity is safe.
- If Blood pressure in range of 180/100 – 199/109. You should consult your doctor before starting any kind of exercise.
- If Blood pressure in range of 200/110 or above. Do not start any exercise without asking your doctor first. You have to take medicine to lower your blood pressure before you can take any kind of exercise.

Specific tips on Exercise with Hypertension.

To keep up healthy heart and control high blood pressure you don't need vigorous exercise. Easy aerobic exercise is enough. Studies show simple exercise such as aerobic exercise if done regularly reduce blood pressure 10 points or more.

Avoid competitive or high-intensity exercises that include bursts of intense exertion. Avoid weights for exercise or use it carefully. Resistance training can lower blood pressure by 2 to 4 percent, but if your blood pressure is 160/100 or more, you should not lift weights. Only if your doctor approves lifting weights, you may do it. If you have your doctor's approval, do one set of 10 to 15 reps using a moderate weight. Try not to hold your breath while lifting, try to exhale when lifting or exerting effort.

After stretching or exercising on the floor, get up slowly. Some blood pressure medications can make you dizzy or sometimes complete black out when you stand or get up quickly. It is called "Orthostatic Hypotension,.." It occurs when blood pressure suddenly drops to a very low pressure with a sudden change of posture.

Skip Caffeine before exercise. A cup of coffee before workout may cause a sudden high in your blood pressure. It is best to avoid caffeine 3 to 4 hours before exercising.

And when working out, remember: always warm up first and cool down after finishing by stretching. This will help your heart to slowly adjust to the activity.

Making exercise a habit can help you continue with the routine. Exercise gives you more energy, and it's a great way to ease stress and feel better. Start by brisk walking, jogging, swimming, biking or doing yard work.

How Often Should You Exercise

Usually, it is best to do a moderate exercise such as walking. Walk for 30 min every day or at least walk 5 days weekly. If you choose more active workout such as jogging, swimming you can work out for 20 minutes at least 5 days. It has the same benefit as 30 min walking.

You can start slow and gradually increase the time. When starting an exercise, warm up for 5 to 10 minutes first to increase your heart rate slowly. Warming up also helps prevent injury. Then, step up the intensity.

When finishing it's best not to stop suddenly. This is especially important if you have high blood pressure. Just slow down for a few minutes. This gives your body a chance to cool down.

When you should stop exercising

If you are starting an exercise with hypertension for the first time, It may take a while before your body gets used to exercise. It is normal to breathe harder and to sweat, it's normal for your heart to beat faster when you're doing exercise.

But if you're feeling very short of breath, or difficulty in breathing or if you feel like your heart is beating too fast or irregularly, stop exercising and rest.

Stop exercising if you feel chest pain, weakness, dizziness, lightheadedness, or pressure or pain in your neck, left arm, left jaw, or left shoulder. If these symptoms continue even after rest, you should consult your doctor.

Manage your weight

Even if you lose only 10% of weight blood pressure is reduced 3 to 4 points

Obesity has become a major health concern worldwide, 65% of adults in the US are overweight. And in case of children aged 2 to 19 one-third of them are obese.

If you are overweight or obese, then weight loss is the most effective lifestyle changes for controlling blood pressure. Even losing a small weight of 10 pounds (4.5 kilograms) can help reduce your blood pressure. One study with 181 overweight and hypertensive patients for 4 years showed that even if you lose only 10% of weight blood pressure is reduced 3 to 4 points.

There are many online calculators available to measure your BMI (Body Mass Index).

You can use the following site to calculate your BMI
https://www.nhlbi.nih.gov/health/educational/lose_wt/BMI/bmicalc.htm

Body mass index (BMI) is an estimation of body fat based on height and weight of adults. BMI between 25 and 30 is considered overweight, over 30 is considered obese. Overweight or Obesity increases load on the heart, blood cholesterol and triglyceride levels increased, and HDL (good) cholesterol levels lower. All of these causes your blood pressure to rise.

Being overweight can also cause disrupted breathing while you sleep, a condition called sleep apnea, which further raises your blood pressure.

Distribution of Fat in your body also has a role. Fat distribution in the abdominal trunk is called abdominal obesity. Abdominal obesity is defined by a waist circumference greater than 102 cm (40in) for men and 88 cm (35 in) for women. Abdominal obesity has the most significant influence on developing hypertension.

Calculate your body mass index and consult your doctor to manage your weight. Use specific diet and exercise recommended by your doctor to lose weight and to control high blood pressure.

Studies show if you lose weight and achieve normal blood pressure you may not need to continue medicine to control your blood pressure. Sometimes if you reach ideal body weight with normal blood pressure, your ongoing medication will be stopped by your doctor.

Alternative ways to reduce high blood pressure
Acupuncture for Hypertension

Acupuncture is a 3000 years old treatment practice originating from China. It is used for treating many diseases.

Usually, Acupuncture is not used as a treatment of Hypertension. In specific situations, you may try acupuncture with the supervision of your doctor or licensed acupuncture professional.

Acupuncture is a 3000 years old treatment practice originating from China. It is used for treating many diseases. In Europe, Canada and western world treatment using acupuncture started 100 years ago, but it becomes popular and widespread rapidly in the second half of the twentieth century. In 1996 US regulators approved acupuncture as a treatment by licensed professionals. According to World Health Organization(WHO), acupuncture is effective for treatment of 28 conditions. Mild to moderate Hypertension can be treated with acupuncture.

Traditional Chinese medicine and acupuncture explain that "Health is the harmonious balance of YIN and YANG. It is believed imbalance between Yin and Yang causes diseases. According to Chinese medicine, our life force is CHI, and it floats through our body via specific points called meridians. Through 350 meridian points of the body, we can access this life force. If acupuncture needle is inserted at specific meridian points, it can restore the balance of Yin and Yang. By restoring balance acupuncture cure diseases.

The medical community throughout the world does not agree on how acupuncture works. By western practitioner, the meridian points are seen as nerve ending, muscle or connective tissue. By acupuncture needle, these nerves or tissue can be stimulated. Which in turn increase blood flow to the area. Acupuncture creates nerve impulse causing painkiller effect or other effects to cure the disease.

On the effect of acupuncture on hypertension, very few studies are done. There is a small study conducted at the University of California Irvine(UCI) on the effect of acupuncture on hypertension. The study shows 70% of the study group shows a noticeable drop in blood pressure. On average systolic blood pressure dropped 6 to 8 mm/Hg, and 4 mm/Hg drop occurred in diastolic blood pressure. And these improvements were persistent for 6 weeks after the treatment. Noradrenaline a hormone and Renin, an enzyme of our body, causes high blood pressure. Acupuncture also shows 4% drop in noradrenalin and a 67% drop in renin.

According to study reduction of high blood pressure were clinically significant and useful for patients 60 or more years of age with systolic hypertension (age-related hypertension).

Risk factors of Acupuncture

- The risk of complication from acupuncture is low. But you must seek a certified acupuncture practitioner. Some complication such as Soreness, Minor bleeding, can occur.
- There is a chance of injury to internal organs such as lungs, heart or spinal cord but it's exceedingly rare.
- You can get infected if the needles are not properly sterilized. There is a chance of transmission of disease such as Hepatitis B or C, HIV etc.

In some condition acupuncture, should not be done

- If you have any type of bleeding disorder, you should not try acupuncture. There is some medicine used in thinning of

blood such as Warfarin causes prolonged bleeding, so acupuncture is contraindicated.
- If you have a pacemaker, then do not try acupuncture especially acupuncture with an electric impulse.
- If you are pregnant acupuncture is contraindicated.

Natural or Herbal Remedies for Hypertension

You will find literally thousand home remedies for Hypertension. There are many medicinal plants used as herbal or natural medicine controlling high blood pressure throughout the world. The problem with home remedies or herbal treatment is that most of the home remedies or herbal treatment has no study or data or has very small study to back up their claims. Study and research are still ongoing to evaluate most of the herbal remedies.

There is a common belief or myth that herbal medicine or Home remedies do not have any side effects or they are safer than other treatment. It's not entirely accurate. To find out the side effect or adverse effect of any medicine we need large studies over a long period but most of the herbal remedies have no proper study. Following herbal remedies need more study before labeling them as safe from side effects;

Rauwolfia serpentina (snakeroot)

Stephania tetrahedra (tetrandrine)

Panax notoginseng (ginseng)

Crataegus species (hawthorn)

Some herbal treatment has proven toxic effect on liver (Hepatotoxic) and Kidneys(Nephrotoxic) in large doses.

Some study shows that following herbal remedies may increase blood pressure, so if you have hypertension, you need to avoid them.

Licorice

Yohimbine

Ephedra (Ma Huang)

Because of potential health risks associated with these herbs, it is important that you inform your doctor if you plan to use or are already using herbal treatment. When some of these herbs are used in combination with high blood pressure drugs it may potentiate or reduce the effects of medicine. They may increase the side effects of drugs when used together.

Following are some home or natural remedies that can lower your blood pressure. There are studies to prove the consequences of these natural remedies.

Hibiscus Tea for High Blood Pressure

Drinking three cups of herbal tea containing hibiscus each day lowered systolic blood pressure by an average of 7 points.

Hibiscus is a beautiful tropical plant. Its scientific name is Hibiscus sabdariffa. Hibiscus tea is prepared by using parts of the hibiscus plant mainly the flower. Hibiscus flowers have various local names, "Roselle" is another commonly used name of hibiscus. Most of the commercial herbal tea blends in the United States contain hibiscus.

Hibiscus tea is used to lower high blood pressure throughout the world. It is a popular medicinal drink preferred by natural medicine practitioners. It contains anthocyanins in high concentration. Anthocyanins inhibit angiotensin-converting enzyme (ACE) and in turn lower blood pressure. The claim is yet to be proved by large study.

There are some small studies done on hibiscus tea. These studies show hibiscus tea lower high blood pressure. One of the studies is done by Diane L. McKay, Ph.D., of Tufts University in Boston. The study shows, "drinking three cups of herbal tea containing hibiscus each day lowered systolic blood pressure by an average of 7 points. That was significantly more than the 1 point drop observed in people who were given hibiscus-flavored water as placebo".

In general, Hibiscus is safe. You can take it as a drink in adequate amount. But it is Unsafe during pregnancy. There is evidence that hibiscus might cause a miscarriage. Based on the research held at the Guru Jambheshwar University of Science and Technology in India. One study concluded that "excessive consumption of hibiscus tea reduces women fertility and effects childbearing. Hibiscus tea might reduce the level of estrogen and affect women's reproductive ability". So, if you are women avoid hibiscus or herbal tea containing hibiscus completely, there is another safe alternative available. There is not enough reliable information or study on the safety of taking hibiscus while breastfeeding. To stay on the safe side, and avoid it during breastfeeding.

Hibiscus might decrease blood sugar levels. Keep monitoring your blood glucose when taking hibiscus tea. If there is frequent low blood sugar, then you need to adjust the dose of your diabetes medications. It is best to consult your doctor.

Garlic for Hypertension

If you want to avoid hypertension drugs, then you should try Garlic first

Garlic is scientifically known as Allium sativum, it is a plant species in the onion group. Garlic is extensively used as natural medicine thousands of years. It is used to treat various diseases or condition in India, China and Egypt, also in Germany and in countries all over the world even where garlic is not readily available.

Medicinal use of garlic has various applications. But it's mostly used in cardiovascular conditions such as Hypertension and heart attack, and to control high levels of fat (Lipids) in your blood called hyperlipidemia.

Research shows that when garlic is taken by mouth for a few months, it can reduce blood pressure by as much as 7% or 8% in people with moderately high blood pressure.

A 2013 meta-analysis study concluded that "garlic preparations may effectively lower total cholesterol by 11–23 mg/dL and LDL cholesterol by 3–15 mg/dL in adults with high cholesterol if taken for longer than two months". By reducing cholesterol, garlic helps to prevent complications of high blood pressure.

Garlic contains a biologically active substance called allicin and garlic sulfides. Garlic works by three mechanisms. Allicin of garlic relaxes blood vessels, maintains a smooth flow lowering blood pressure and vessel damage. It also blocks the function of angiotensin (angiotensin is responsible for raising blood pressure) to keep blood vessels relaxed and wide. Garlic also activates the production of nitric oxide synthesis which helps relax blood vessels.

If you want to control blood pressure with natural products, if you want to avoid hypertension drugs then you should try Garlic first. Most likely it will lower blood pressure to a normal level.

Garlic is safe for most people when taken by mouth appropriately and in a small amount, It can be taken for a long time. Garlic has been used safely in research for up to 7 years without any side effect.

There are some minor side effects in some people. When taken by mouth, garlic can cause

Burning sensation in the mouth or stomach.

- Heartburn.
- Abdominal bloating.
- Sometimes nausea, vomiting, and diarrhea.

These side effects are often worse with raw garlic. If you experience any of these, you may switch to Garlic Capsule available over the counter.

Garlic is known to cause bad breath (halitosis) and body odor, a pungent "garlicky" smell to sweat. This is caused by allyl methyl sulfide (AMS) present in garlic.

AMS is a volatile liquid which is absorbed into the blood from the stomach. Then via blood, it travels to the lungs. As it is a volatile substance, it is expelled by respiration causing bad breath. Some garlic products are made "odorless" by aging the garlic, but this makes garlic less effective. You may take supplements that are coated, so they dissolve in the intestine instead of stomach.

If you want to try garlic be sure to consult your partner first. Your partner will be suffered from your bad breath and garlicky body odor!

For individual dose consult your doctor.

Food supplements for hypertension

Certain food supplements can lower blood pressure. Most of the supplements show promising results in studies.

Coenzyme Q10 (CoQ10)

Coenzyme Q10 is a naturally occurring enzyme in our body. Studies at the University of Texas and in Osaka, Japan, showed very promising result in controlling hypertension. It showed that if 45 to 60 mg of CoQ10 is taken daily, it lowered blood pressure levels 12 to 25 points or more. In the study, patients with moderate high blood pressure taking CoQ10 alone without any medicine reduced blood pressure to a normal level.

Coenzyme Q10 has other beneficial effects. It helps maintain circulatory health by keeping heart muscle and blood vessels healthy.

Omega-3 fatty acids

you should eat fish (particularly fatty, cold water fish) at least twice a week

There are some nutritional substance essential for us but our body is unable to make them. They are called essential fatty acids. As our body, can't make them we have to get it from our diet. Omega-3 fatty acid is one of these essential fatty acids.

Several clinical studies show that Omega-3 has a positive effect on heart and blood vessels. It also lowers blood pressure in hypertensive patients. An analysis of 17 clinical studies using fish oil supplements as a source of Omega-3, found that taking fish rich in omega-3 daily reduce blood pressure in people with hypertension.

Modest reductions in blood pressure occur with a significantly higher dose of 3 or more grams of omega-3 fatty acids. But more than 3 gm of Omega 3 increase the risk of bleeding. So don't take more than 3 gm.

The American Heart Association (AHA) recommends that "you should eat fish (particularly fatty, cold water fish) at least twice a week." Other fishes containing a rich source of Omega-3 are Salmon, mackerel, herring, sardines, lake trout, and tuna. The AHA says taking up to 3 or less than 3 grams of fish oil daily in supplement form is safe and beneficial.

Side effects from omega-3 fish oil may include:

- A fishy taste in your mouth
- Fishy breath
- Abdominal distension and discomfort
- Loose stools
- Nausea

Meditation for Hypertension

Prayer is a powerful form of meditation.

Anxiety, stress or tension not only cause a sudden increase in blood pressure it has a lasting effect. During stress, a hormone called Adrenaline gets released and the level of adrenaline increases in our body. Adrenaline increase the heart rate leading to raised blood pressure. Anxiety and stress are also responsible for other dangerous conditions such as stroke and heart attack.

Meditation is a thousand years old practice. We have used meditation since the dawn of medical science developed by shamans. And studies have proven that this ancient treatment works in many conditions. In modern times, new methods of meditation are being developed for specific conditions. For high blood pressure a particular type of meditation called "Transcendental Meditation" works best.

Usually, in meditation, we use a deep breath with focusing on tranquility of mind. It causes a deep relaxation without sleep and removes stress from our mind. Transcend meditation uses deep breathing with a focus on any color or sound or peaceful memory to concentrate.

Recent studies have offered promising results about the impact of Transcend Meditation in reducing blood pressure. A 2012 study (in African American 5 year follow-up) showed that with Transendal Meditation the risk of heart attack or stroke is 48% reduced.

For Transendal meditation you will need a quiet environment. Some soothing music or sound can be used. You can also focus on your heart beat or respiration.

You need to be seated with eyes closed. Concentrate on any music, sound or a peaceful memory. Relax but don't work too hard on focusing. You need to do this for 15 to 20 minutes, best if done twice a day.

Studies have shown meditation is very effective in easing stress. We think the deeply relaxed state of meditation may start biochemical changes beneficial to the body. It may trigger the self-healing capacity of our body. It restores the balance between our mind and body.

There are many types of meditation, so start anything that you are comfortable with. Try some different types of meditation to know what works for you.

A prayer is also a powerful form of meditation.

Simple steps to control your hypertension

Now you have all the information needed to understand hypertension. You should be able to choose the plan that works for you. Following are some simple steps, use them to plan your individualized routine.

- Calculate your BMI and lose weight if your BMI is high. Use specific diet and exercise in combination to maximize weight loss.

- Modify your diet. Eat meals that are high in fiber, minerals, vitamins and low in salt. Take supplements like Omega 3, Coenzyme alternatively every month until you see a significant difference in your blood pressure.

- Exercise at least 4 days every week.

- Meditate at least once every week.

- Spend more time with friends and family and engage in events with friends and relatives at least 3 times every week.

- Read updates on high blood pressure once every week to keep yourself motivated.

Conclusion

High blood pressure, leading to the life-threatening complication is a reality. All the study and data indicate that most of us will get high blood pressure. So, you need to be prepared and start preventive measure as early as possible. I hope after reading this book, you can choose a plan that works for you.

Always remember high blood pressure or hypertension is easy to control. And with minimal effort, you can Prevent Hypertension.

THE END

Other Books by Dr. Shahriar Mostafa

Diagnosed with Diabetes. Now What!
Smallest Book with Everything You Need to Know

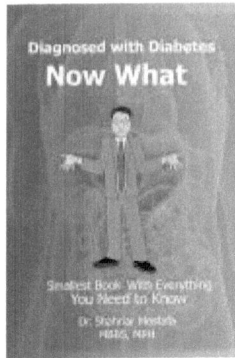

You were living your life to the fullest. Working hard and playing harder. Ignoring symptoms like fatigue, weight loss and increased frequency of urination. Then BAM! Out of the blue you started feeling very sick. You consult with your doctor, he runs some tests and you are diagnosed with diabetes!
Now What!

Should you leave all the things you love to do? Stop eating desserts. Adopt a life of Saints! Should you get panicked and think that's it, this is the end of the road! Well, it's not like that.

This book will help you to keep your diabetes well controlled. It's a small book but packed with information on diabetes you must know. Grab your copy and let's start for a healthy, happy and fulfilling life with Diabetes.

Type One Diabetes:
Smallest book with everything you need to know

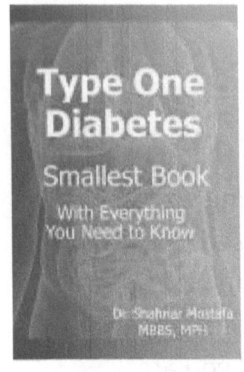

As soon as you learn that you or your child has type one diabetes you become terrified. What happens in type one diabetes? What to do to cure it? How to control it? How to explain this to a child? What's causing it? Why did it happen to me? Thousand and thousand questions pop up in your mind. You search the internet which shows a million pages. You ask your health care personal but not satisfied with the answers. You become confused, afraid and angry.

But you don't have to be confused or afraid. You are not alone. Type one diabetes is a common disease. About 350 million people worldwide have diabetes. It is easy to control. It does not keep you from anything the life has to offer. But there is a catch, you have to control type one diabetes all your life.

Type 2 Diabetes:
Smallest book with everything you need to know

Diabetes is a common disease. About 350 million people worldwide have diabetes. It is easy to control. It does not keep you from anything the life has to offer. But there is a catch, you have to control Diabetes all your life.

This book is small and you do not have to read this book from page one to the end. You can start anywhere and slowly finish it. Use the table of contents to find the topic of your interest and start from there. You can finish this book in just 1 hour. In 1 hour, you will have all important information on Type 2 Diabetes. This book will give the confidence, hope and information to live a normal, happy life with Type 2 Diabetes.

Pregnancy & Diabetes:
Smallest Book with Everything You need to know

If you are pregnant or planning for pregnancy, congratulations. Pregnancy is a life changing event. It takes a lot of courage and a lot more love to make a decision to have a baby. A lot of planning is also needed before, during and after the pregnancy. Most of us never think twice about diabetes, unless we have it. But diabetes specifically gestational diabetes is a major concern during pregnancy, even if you do not have diabetes.

www.ingramcontent.com/pod-product-compliance
Lightning Source LLC
Chambersburg PA
CBHW020929180526
45163CB00007B/2940